HAND REFLEXOLOGY
COMPENDIUM

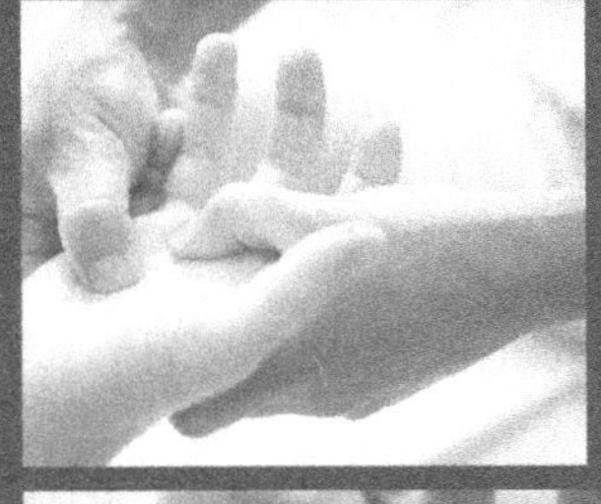
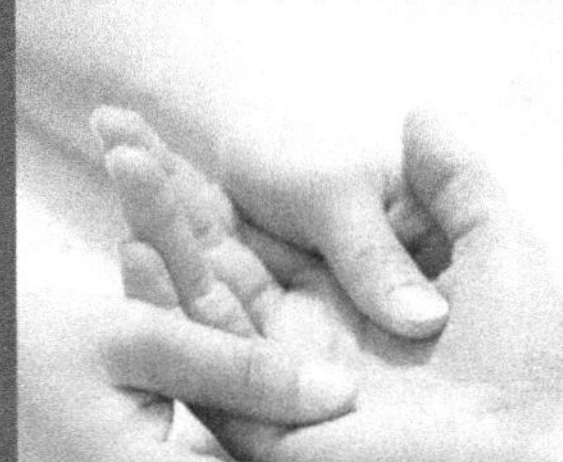
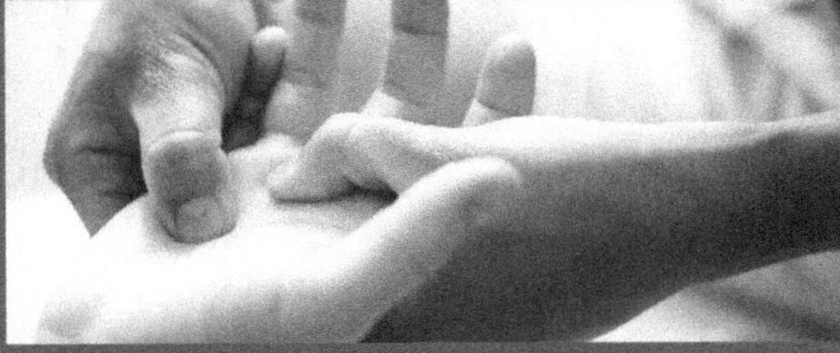

Dr. James K. Ferguson

COPYRIGHT © 2024 by Dr. James K. Ferguson

TABLE OF CONTENTS

TABLE OF CONTENTS ---------------------- 2-5

INTRODUCTION ------------------------------ 6-9

CHAPTER 1 ------------------------------------ 10-15

20 important things you should know about Hand Reflexology

CHAPTER 2 ---------------------------------- 16-29

Overview of Hand Reflexology

Benefits of Hand Reflexology

How Hand Reflexology Works

History of Hand Reflexology

CHAPTER 3 ---------------------------------- 30-47

Understanding the Basics of Hand Reflexology

Principles of Reflexology

Zones and Points on the Hands in Reflexology

Techniques Used in Hand Reflexology

Tools and Accessories for Hand Reflexology

CHAPTER 4 ---------------------------------- 48-64

Getting Started with Hand Reflexology

Preparing for a Hand Reflexology Session

Setting the Right Environment for Hand Reflexology

Techniques for Relaxation in Hand Reflexology

CHAPTER 5 ————————————————————— 65-76

Mapping the Hand

How to Locate Reflex Points on the Hands

Understanding the Connection between Hands and Body in Reflexology

CHAPTER 6 ————————————————————— 77-92

Practicing Hand Reflexology

Step-by-Step Guide to Performing Hand Reflexology

Common Hand Reflexology Techniques

Tips for Effective Hand Reflexology Sessions

CHAPTER 7 ————————————————————— 93-107

Hand Reflexology for Specific Conditions

Using Hand Reflexology for Pain Relief

Hand Reflexology for Stress and Anxiety Relief

Hand Reflexology for Better Sleep

CHAPTER 8 ————————————————————— 108-121

Incorporating Hand Reflexology into Your Wellness Routine

Integrating Hand Reflexology with Other Wellness Practices

Daily Hand Reflexology Exercises for Self-Care

Maintaining Hand Health for Reflexology

CHAPTER 9 ———————————————————————— 122-137

Advanced Hand Reflexology Techniques

Advanced Hand Reflexology Points and Zones

Reflexology for Emotional Wellbeing through the Hands

Hand Reflexology for Energy Balance

CHAPTER 10 ——————————————————————— 138-152

Exploring Reflexology Traditions

Different Traditions and Approaches to Hand Reflexology

Cultural and Historical Perspectives on Hand Reflexology

Modern Innovations in Hand Reflexology

CHAPTER 11 ——————————————————————— 153-169

Frequently Asked Questions about Hand Reflexology

Addressing Common Concerns and Misconceptions about Hand Reflexology

Tips for Enhancing Your Hand Reflexology Practice

Troubleshooting Issues during Hand Reflexology Sessions

CHAPTER 12 ——————————————————————— 170-177

The Future of Hand Reflexology

Final Thoughts and Encouragement for Practitioners of Hand Reflexology

CHAPTER 13 ------------------------------- 178-185

Key Terms and Concepts in Hand Reflexology

Comprehensive Index of Topics Covered in the "Hand Reflexology Compendium "

CONCLUSION ---------------------------- 186-188

INTRODUCTION

Welcome to the world of hand reflexology, where the key to your well-being lies literally at your fingertips. In this comprehensive guide, we explore the ancient practice of reflexology, focusing specifically on the hands, a powerful yet often overlooked gateway to holistic health.

Imagine a world where you can alleviate stress, relieve pain, and promote healing without medication or invasive procedures. Hand reflexology offers just that, a natural, non-invasive approach to health and wellness that anyone can learn and practice.

Embark on a Journey of Discovery: In "Hand Reflexology Compendium ," it starts with the 20 important things everyone should know about hand reflexology, principles, techniques, and benefits of hand reflexology, providing you with the knowledge and tools to unlock the healing potential of your hands. Whether you are new to reflexology or an experienced practitioner, this book offers something for everyone.

Understanding the Basics: Begin by laying the foundation, explaining the principles of reflexology, the zones and points on the hands, and the techniques used in hand reflexology. You'll learn how to prepare for a hand reflexology session, set the right environment, and techniques for relaxation.

Mapping the Hands: Next, together we dive into the intricate map of the hands, detailing the reflex points and their corresponding body parts.

You'll discover how to locate these points on your hands and understand the profound connection between your hands and your body.

Practicing Hand Reflexology: With step-by-step instructions, accompanied by illustrations, you'll learn how to perform hand reflexology on yourself and others. From basic techniques to advanced practices, this book guides you through each step, ensuring you get the most out of your reflexology sessions.

Unlock the Healing Power of Your Hands: By incorporating hand reflexology into your wellness routine, you'll not only improve your physical health but also enhance your emotional well-being and energy balance. Discover how daily hand reflexology exercises can become a powerful tool for self-care and healing.

As you embark on this journey of self-discovery and healing, remember that the power to heal lies within you. Your hands are not just instruments for daily tasks, they are powerful tools for promoting health, relieving stress, and enhancing your overall well-being. Take the first step towards a healthier, more balanced life, dive into the world of hand reflexology and unlock the healing power of your hands.

CHAPTER 1

20 Important things you should know about Hand Reflexology

1. Hand reflexology is a holistic therapy that involves applying pressure to specific points on the hands to promote healing and relaxation in corresponding areas of the body.

2. Like foot reflexology, hand reflexology is based on the principle that there are reflex points on the hands that correspond to different organs, glands, and parts of the body.

3. Hand reflexology is believed to help improve circulation, reduce tension, and promote a sense of well-being.

4. This therapy can be used to address a wide range of health issues, including stress, anxiety, headaches, and digestive problems.

5. Hand reflexology is a non-invasive therapy that is generally safe for most people, although it may not be suitable for those with certain hand conditions or medical issues.

6. A hand reflexology session typically lasts between 15 and 30 minutes and can be a relaxing and rejuvenating experience.

7. Regular hand reflexology sessions may help improve overall health and well-being by promoting relaxation and reducing stress.

8. Hand reflexology is suitable for people of all ages, from children to the elderly.

9. It is important to choose a qualified and experienced reflexologist when seeking hand reflexology treatment.

10. Hand reflexology is not a substitute for medical care, and it is important to consult with a healthcare professional for any serious health concerns.

11. Some people may experience discomfort during a hand reflexology session, but this is usually temporary and should subside quickly.

12. Hand reflexology can be a beneficial therapy for those looking to improve their overall health and well-being in a natural and holistic way.

13. The practice of hand reflexology has been used for thousands of years in various cultures around the world.

14. Hand reflexology is believed to help balance the body's energy and promote a sense of harmony and well-being.

15. Some research suggests that hand reflexology may be effective in reducing pain and improving quality of life for people with certain health conditions.

16. Hand reflexology can be a cost-effective and non-invasive way to improve your health and well-being.

17. Many people find that hand reflexology helps them feel more relaxed and rejuvenated, with improved hand flexibility and function.

18. Hand reflexology can be easily incorporated into your daily self-care routine for added benefits.

19. Overall, hand reflexology is a safe and effective therapy that can help improve your health and well-being in a natural and holistic way.

20. Learning and practicing hand reflexology can be a rewarding experience, providing you with valuable self-care tools for life.

CHAPTER 2

Overview of Hand Reflexology

Hand reflexology is a holistic healing technique that involves applying pressure to specific points on the hands to promote relaxation, relieve stress, and stimulate healing in corresponding parts of the body. It is based on the principle that there are reflex points on the hands that are connected to different organs and systems in the body through energy channels.

This ancient practice has been used for centuries in various cultures around the world as a natural way to improve health and well-being. Hand reflexology is believed to help balance the body's energy flow, improve circulation, and enhance the body's natural ability to heal itself.

One of the key benefits of hand reflexology is its accessibility. Unlike foot reflexology, which requires removing footwear and exposing the feet, hand reflexology can be done anywhere, anytime, making it a convenient option for self-care and relaxation.

Hand reflexology is often used as a complementary therapy to support conventional medical treatments. It is commonly used to alleviate symptoms of stress, anxiety, and pain, as well as to improve circulation and promote overall wellness.

Practicing hand reflexology involves using various techniques, such as thumb-walking, finger-walking, and kneading, to apply pressure to specific points on the hands. These points correspond to different organs and systems in the body, and by stimulating these points, practitioners believe they can help restore balance and harmony to the body.

Overall, hand reflexology is a gentle, non-invasive therapy that can be a valuable tool for promoting health and well-being. It is suitable for people of all ages and can be easily incorporated into a daily self-care routine to help maintain optimal health.

Benefits of Hand Reflexology

Hand reflexology offers a myriad of benefits that can positively impact both physical and mental health. This ancient practice is believed to stimulate the body's natural healing processes, promote relaxation, and improve overall well-being.

Some of the key benefits of hand reflexology include:

1. Stress Relief: One of the most well-known benefits of hand reflexology is its ability to induce relaxation and reduce stress. By applying pressure to specific points on the hands, this technique can help calm the mind and body, leading to a sense of peace and tranquility.

2. Pain Management: Hand reflexology has been shown to be effective in managing various types of pain, including headaches, back pain, and arthritis. By targeting specific reflex points on the hands, this technique can help alleviate pain and discomfort, promoting a greater sense of well-being.

3. Improved Circulation: The stimulation of reflex points on the hands during hand reflexology can help improve blood circulation. This can have a range of benefits, including better oxygenation of tissues, improved nutrient delivery, and enhanced waste removal from the body.

4. Enhanced Immune Function: Hand reflexology is believed to support the immune system by helping to remove blockages in the body's energy pathways. By promoting balance and harmony within the body, hand reflexology may help strengthen the immune system and improve overall health.

5. Relaxation and Better Sleep: Regular practice of hand reflexology can promote relaxation and improve sleep quality. By reducing stress and tension, hand reflexology can help individuals achieve a state of deep relaxation, leading to better sleep patterns and improved overall health.

6. Emotional Well-being: Hand reflexology is not only beneficial for physical health but can also have a positive impact on emotional well-being. By promoting relaxation and reducing stress, hand reflexology can help improve mood and promote a sense of overall happiness and well-being.

7. Complementary Therapy: Hand reflexology is often used as a complementary therapy alongside conventional medical treatments. It can be used to support individuals with various health conditions, helping to improve their overall quality of life.

In summary, hand reflexology offers a range of benefits for both the body and mind. By incorporating this ancient practice into your daily routine, you can experience improved health, reduced stress, and a greater sense of well-being.

How Hand Reflexology Works

Hand reflexology is based on the principle that there are reflex points on the hands that correspond to specific organs, glands, and other parts of the body. By applying pressure to these reflex points, practitioners believe they can stimulate the body's natural healing processes and promote overall health and well-being.

1. Reflex Zones on the Hands: The hands are divided into various reflex zones, each corresponding to a different part of the body. For example, the tips of the fingers are believed to correspond to the head and neck, while the base of the fingers corresponds to the chest and lungs.

2. Stimulating Reflex Points: During a hand reflexology session, the practitioner will apply pressure to specific reflex points on the hands using their fingers, thumbs, and palms. This pressure is applied in a rhythmic and controlled manner, and can vary in intensity depending on the individual's needs.

3. Energy Flow: Practitioners of hand reflexology believe that by applying pressure to the reflex points, they can help to unblock or balance the flow of energy, known as qi or chi, through the body. This, in turn, is believed to promote healing and improve overall health.

4. Nerve Stimulation: The pressure applied during hand reflexology is also thought to stimulate the nerves in the hands, which can have a positive impact on the corresponding areas of the body. This stimulation is believed to help reduce pain, improve circulation, and enhance overall well-being.

5. Relaxation Response: One of the key benefits of hand reflexology is its ability to induce a state of relaxation. The pressure applied to the reflex points can help to calm the nervous system, reduce stress, and promote a sense of peace and tranquility.

6. Holistic Approach: Hand reflexology is considered a holistic therapy, meaning it treats the whole person, not just the symptoms of a particular ailment. By promoting balance and harmony within the body, hand reflexology aims to support overall health and well-being.

In summary, hand reflexology works by stimulating specific reflex points on the hands to promote healing, reduce stress, and improve overall health. This ancient practice offers a natural, non-invasive approach to wellness that can be easily incorporated into your daily routine.

History of Hand Reflexology

Hand reflexology is a practice that has been around for centuries, with roots in ancient healing traditions from various cultures around the world. The concept of reflexology, which includes hand reflexology, is based on the idea that there are reflex points on the hands, feet, and other parts of the body that correspond to specific organs, glands, and body systems.

Ancient Origins: The origins of hand reflexology can be traced back to ancient Egypt, China, and India, where it was practiced as a form of natural healing. Ancient Egyptian hieroglyphics depict scenes of foot and hand massage, suggesting that reflexology was used to treat various ailments.

Chinese Reflexology: In Chinese medicine, the hands are considered to be a mirror of the body, with each part of the hand corresponding to a different organ or body system. Chinese reflexology, which includes hand reflexology, is based on the principle that stimulating these reflex points can help to restore balance and harmony within the body.

European Influence: Hand reflexology gained popularity in Europe during the 19th century, particularly in countries such as Germany and Russia. It was during this time that the modern concept of reflexology, as we know it today, began to take shape.

Modern Development: In the early 20th century, American physiotherapist Eunice Ingham further developed the practice of reflexology, focusing specifically on the feet. She mapped out the reflex points on the feet and developed techniques for stimulating these points to promote healing and relieve pain.

Popularity Today: Today, hand reflexology is practiced around the world as a form of complementary therapy. It is often used alongside conventional medical treatments to support overall health and well-being. Hand reflexology is popular due to its accessibility and ease of practice, making it a convenient option for self-care and relaxation.

Hand reflexology has a rich history that spans across cultures and centuries. Its popularity continues to grow as more people discover its potential benefits for health and well-being. Whether used as a standalone therapy or as part of a holistic approach to health, hand reflexology offers a natural and effective way to promote healing and enhance overall wellness.

CHAPTER 3

Understanding the Basics of Hand Reflexology

Hand reflexology is a holistic healing technique that involves applying pressure to specific points on the hands to promote relaxation, relieve stress, and stimulate healing in corresponding parts of the body. This practice is based on the belief that the hands contain reflex points that are connected to different organs and systems in the body through energy channels.

Principles of Hand Reflexology: The practice of hand reflexology is based on several key principles. One of the fundamental principles is that the body is reflected in a microcosm on the hands, with each part of the hand corresponding to a specific organ or body system. By stimulating these reflex points, practitioners believe they can help to restore balance and harmony within the body.

Zones and Points on the Hands: The hands are divided into various zones and points, each of which corresponds to a different part of the body. For example, the tips of the fingers are believed to correspond to the head and neck, while the base of the fingers corresponds to the chest and lungs.

Techniques Used in Hand Reflexology: Hand reflexology involves using various techniques to apply pressure to the reflex points on the hands. Common techniques include thumb-walking, finger-walking, and kneading. These techniques are designed to stimulate the reflex points and promote healing responses in the corresponding areas of the body.

Tools and Accessories: While hand reflexology can be practiced using just the hands, some practitioners may use tools or accessories to enhance the practice. These may include hand reflexology charts, which map out the reflex points on the hands, or essential oils, which can be used to enhance relaxation and promote healing.

Benefits of Hand Reflexology: Hand reflexology offers a range of benefits, including stress relief, pain management, improved circulation, and enhanced immune function. It is also believed to promote relaxation and emotional well-being.

In summary, hand reflexology is a gentle and non-invasive therapy that can be used to promote health and well-being. By understanding the basics of hand reflexology, you can incorporate this ancient practice into your daily routine to support your overall health and vitality.

Principles of Reflexology

Reflexology is based on the principle that there are reflex points on the hands, feet, and ears that correspond to specific organs, glands, and other parts of the body. By stimulating these reflex points, practitioners believe they can promote healing, reduce stress, and restore balance within the body.

The principles of reflexology include:

1. Zones and Reflex Points: Reflexologists divide the body into ten longitudinal zones, five on each side of the body. Each zone corresponds to specific areas on the hands, feet, and ears. Reflex points are specific points within these zones that correspond to different parts of the body.

2. Holistic Approach: Reflexology is based on the principle that the body is interconnected, and that imbalances in one part of the body can affect other parts. By working on the reflex points, reflexologists aim to restore balance and harmony within the body as a whole.

3. Energy Flow: Reflexologists believe that there is a flow of energy, or life force, throughout the body. This energy can become blocked or stagnant, leading to illness or discomfort. By stimulating the reflex points, reflexologists aim to clear blockages and restore the smooth flow of energy.

4. Reflexology Maps: Reflexologists use maps or charts that show the location of reflex points on the hands, feet, and ears. These maps help practitioners identify the reflex points that correspond to specific organs or body systems.

5. Relaxation and Healing Response: One of the main goals of reflexology is to induce a state of deep relaxation, which can help the body heal itself. Reflexology is believed to stimulate the release of endorphins, the body's natural painkillers, and promote a sense of well-being.

6. Complementary Therapy: Reflexology is often used as a complementary therapy alongside conventional medical treatments. It is not intended to replace medical care, but rather to support and enhance the body's natural healing processes.

In summary, reflexology is a holistic therapy based on the principle that there are reflex points on the hands, feet, and ears that correspond to different parts of the body. By stimulating these reflex points, reflexologists aim to promote healing, reduce stress, and restore balance within the body.

Zones and Points on the Hands in Reflexology

In reflexology, the hands are divided into zones and points that correspond to different parts of the body. These zones and points are believed to be connected through energy channels, and by stimulating them, practitioners aim to promote healing and restore balance within the body. **Here is an overview of the zones and points on the hands:**

1. Thumb Zone: The thumb zone corresponds to the head and neck area. The tip of the thumb is believed to correspond to the brain, while the base of the thumb corresponds to the neck.

2. Index Finger Zone: The index finger zone corresponds to the digestive and respiratory systems. The tip of the index finger is believed to correspond to the sinuses, while the base of the index finger corresponds to the lungs and bronchi.

3. Middle Finger Zone: The middle finger zone corresponds to the circulatory and nervous systems. The tip of the middle finger is believed to correspond to the heart, while the base of the middle finger corresponds to the upper back and spine.

4. Ring Finger Zone: The ring finger zone corresponds to the reproductive and endocrine systems. The tip of the ring finger is believed to correspond to the reproductive organs, while the base of the ring finger corresponds to the adrenal glands.

5. Little Finger Zone: The little finger zone corresponds to the excretory system and metabolism. The tip of the little finger is believed to correspond to the kidneys, while the base of the little finger corresponds to the lower back and pelvis.

Reflex Points: In addition to the zones, there are specific reflex points on the hands that correspond to different organs and body parts. These points are located in specific areas within each zone and are believed to be connected to the corresponding body parts through energy channels.

Stimulation Techniques: Reflexologists use various techniques to stimulate the reflex points on the hands, including thumb-walking, finger-walking, and kneading. These techniques are designed to apply pressure to the reflex points and promote healing responses in the corresponding areas of the body.

In summary, the zones and points on the hands in reflexology correspond to different parts of the body, and by stimulating these zones and points, practitioners aim to promote healing, reduce stress, and restore balance within the body.

Techniques Used in Hand Reflexology

Hand reflexology involves the application of pressure to specific points on the hands to promote relaxation, relieve stress, and stimulate healing in corresponding parts of the body. There are several techniques used in hand reflexology, each designed to target different reflex points and achieve specific therapeutic effects.

Some of the common techniques used in hand reflexology include:

1. Thumb Walking: This technique involves using the thumb to apply firm but gentle pressure to the reflex points on the hands. The thumb is moved in a walking motion, applying pressure to each point in a systematic manner.

2. Finger Walking: Similar to thumb walking, finger walking involves using the fingers to apply pressure to the reflex points on the hands. The fingers are moved in a walking motion, applying pressure to each point to stimulate the corresponding area of the body.

3. Kneading: Kneading is a technique that involves using the fingers and thumbs to gently knead the reflex points on the hands. This helps to stimulate circulation and promote relaxation in the hands and corresponding areas of the body.

4. Rotational Movements: Rotational movements involve using the fingers or thumbs to make circular motions on the reflex points. This helps to stimulate the reflex points and promote healing in the corresponding areas of the body.

5. Friction: Friction is a technique that involves rubbing the reflex points on the hands briskly to create heat and stimulate circulation. This can help to relieve tension and promote relaxation in the hands and body.

6. Finger Pressing: Finger pressing involves using the fingers to apply firm pressure to specific reflex points on the hands. This helps to stimulate the reflex points and promote healing in the corresponding areas of the body.

7. Hook and Back-Up: This technique involves using the thumb to hook onto a reflex point and then backing up with the thumb to apply pressure. This can help to stimulate the reflex points and promote healing in the corresponding areas of the body.

These techniques are just a few examples of the many methods used in hand reflexology. By applying pressure to specific points on the hands, practitioners aim to stimulate the body's natural healing processes and promote overall health and well-being. Whether used as a standalone therapy or as part of a holistic approach to health, hand reflexology offers a natural and effective way to support your body's healing abilities.

Tools and Accessories for Hand Reflexology

While hand reflexology can be practiced using just the hands, there are several tools and accessories that can enhance the practice and improve its effectiveness. These tools and accessories can help practitioners locate reflex points more easily, apply pressure more effectively, and enhance the overall experience of hand reflexology.

Some common tools and accessories used in hand reflexology include:

1. Reflexology Charts: Reflexology charts are diagrams that show the reflex points on the hands and feet, as well as their corresponding body parts. These charts can be used as a reference guide to help practitioners locate the reflex points and target them more effectively during a reflexology session.

2. Essential Oils: Essential oils are often used in hand reflexology to enhance relaxation and promote healing. Certain essential oils, such as lavender and chamomile, are known for their calming and soothing properties, making them ideal for use in reflexology sessions.

3. Hand Cream or Massage Oil: Hand cream or massage oil can be used to lubricate the hands during a reflexology session, making it easier to apply pressure to the reflex points. Additionally, the moisturizing properties of hand cream or massage oil can help to soften the skin and enhance the overall experience of hand reflexology.

4. Hand Massager: A hand massager is a tool that can be used to apply pressure to the reflex points on the hands. Hand massagers come in a variety of shapes and sizes, and can be used to target specific reflex points or provide a more general massage of the hands.

5. Hand Roller: A hand roller is a small, handheld tool that can be used to apply pressure to the reflex points on the hands. Hand rollers typically have a textured surface that helps to stimulate the reflex points and promote healing.

6. Acupressure Rings: Acupressure rings are small, metal rings that can be worn on the fingers during a reflexology session. The rings have small, raised points that apply pressure to the reflex points on the hands, helping to stimulate circulation and promote healing.

These tools and accessories can help enhance the practice of hand reflexology, making it more effective and enjoyable for both practitioners and clients. Whether used alone or in combination, these tools can help to improve the overall experience of hand reflexology and promote better health and well-being.

CHAPTER 4

Getting Started with Hand Reflexology

Hand reflexology is a simple and effective way to promote relaxation, relieve stress, and support overall health and well-being. Whether you're new to reflexology or an experienced practitioner, here are some steps to help you get started with hand reflexology:

1. Learn the Basics: Begin by familiarizing yourself with the basic principles of hand reflexology. Learn about the zones and reflex points on the hands, and how they correspond to different organs and body systems.

2. Gather Your Tools: While hand reflexology can be practiced using just the hands, you may want to consider using tools and accessories such as reflexology charts, essential oils, hand cream, or a hand massager to enhance your practice.

3. Set the Mood: Create a relaxing environment for your hand reflexology session. Choose a quiet and comfortable space where you won't be disturbed, and consider playing soft music or lighting candles to create a calming atmosphere.

4. Prepare Your Hands: Wash your hands thoroughly with warm water and soap to clean them and relax the muscles. Dry your hands thoroughly before beginning your session.

5. Start with Relaxation Techniques: Begin your hand reflexology session by using gentle techniques to relax the hands. You can use kneading, circular motions, or simply hold the hand and apply gentle pressure to help your client relax.

6. Locate the Reflex Points: Use a reflexology chart as a guide to locate the reflex points on the hands. Apply pressure to these points using your thumb, fingers, or a hand massager, using a firm but gentle touch.

7. Use a Systematic Approach: Work on one hand at a time, starting with the thumb and working your way down to the little finger. Apply pressure to each reflex point in a systematic manner, focusing on areas that correspond to any specific issues or concerns.

8. Practice Regularly: To experience the full benefits of hand reflexology, practice regularly. Aim for at least 10-15 minutes per hand, several times a week, to promote relaxation, relieve stress, and support overall health and well-being.

By following these simple steps, you can begin to enjoy the many benefits of hand reflexology. Whether you're looking to relax after a long day or support your overall health, hand reflexology is a gentle and effective way to promote wellness for both body and mind.

Preparing for a Hand Reflexology Session

Preparing for a hand reflexology session involves creating a relaxing environment and ensuring that both the practitioner and the client are comfortable.

Here are some steps to help you prepare for a hand reflexology session:

1. Set the Mood: Choose a quiet and comfortable space for the reflexology session. Dim the lights, play soft music, and use aromatherapy diffusers or candles with relaxing scents such as lavender or chamomile to create a calming atmosphere.

2. Gather Your Supplies: Have all the necessary tools and accessories ready, including reflexology charts, essential oils, hand cream or massage oil, and any other tools you plan to use during the session.

3. Prepare the Hands: Wash your hands thoroughly with warm water and soap to clean them and relax the muscles. Dry your hands thoroughly before beginning the session.

4. Relaxation Techniques: Start the session with relaxation techniques to help the client unwind. You can gently massage the hands or use calming techniques such as breathing exercises to help the client relax.

5. Explain the Process: Before starting the reflexology session, explain the process to the client and answer any questions they may have. Let them know what to expect during the session and how they can benefit from the treatment.

6. Locate the Reflex Points: Use a reflexology chart to locate the reflex points on the hands.

Apply gentle pressure to these points using your thumb, fingers, or a hand massager, focusing on areas that correspond to the client's specific needs.

7. Use a Systematic Approach: Work on one hand at a time, starting with the thumb and working your way down to the little finger. Apply pressure to each reflex point in a systematic manner, taking your time to ensure that you cover all the areas of the hand.

8. Monitor the Client's Response: Pay attention to the client's response during the session. Look for signs of discomfort or tension and adjust your pressure or technique accordingly. Encourage the client to communicate any sensations or feelings they experience during the session.

9. Finish with Relaxation Techniques: Once you have completed the reflexology session, finish with relaxation techniques to help the client transition back to a state of wakefulness. Gently massage the hands and encourage the client to take a few deep breaths before slowly returning to a seated position.

10. Provide Aftercare Instructions: After the session, provide the client with aftercare instructions, such as drinking plenty of water, avoiding caffeine and alcohol, and practicing self-care techniques at home to prolong the benefits of the reflexology session.

By following these steps, you can ensure that both you and your client are prepared for a hand reflexology session. Creating a relaxing environment and using gentle, systematic techniques can help enhance the effectiveness of the session and promote overall health and well-being.

Setting the Right Environment for Hand Reflexology

Creating the right environment for a hand reflexology session is crucial for promoting relaxation, relieving stress, and enhancing the overall experience for both the practitioner and the client.

Here are some key aspects to consider when setting the environment for a hand reflexology session:

1. Choose a Quiet Space: Select a quiet and peaceful space for the reflexology session.

Ensure that the room is free from distractions and noise, allowing the client to fully relax and unwind.

2. Create a Comfortable Seating Area: Provide a comfortable chair or recliner for the client to sit in during the session. Use cushions or pillows to support the client's back and arms, ensuring they are comfortable throughout the session.

3. Use Soft Lighting: Dim the lights in the room to create a relaxing ambiance. Consider using lamps with soft, warm-toned bulbs or candles to add to the soothing atmosphere.

4. Play Relaxing Music: Choose calming music or nature sounds to play in the background during the session. Soft instrumental music or sounds of nature, such as gentle rain or ocean waves, can help promote relaxation and create a serene environment.

5. Incorporate Aromatherapy: Use essential oils or aromatherapy diffusers to infuse the room with relaxing scents. Lavender, chamomile, and sandalwood are popular choices known for their calming properties.

6. Maintain a Comfortable Temperature: Ensure that the room is at a comfortable temperature for the client. Use blankets or a space heater to adjust the temperature as needed to keep the client warm and comfortable.

7. Create a Relaxing Atmosphere: Consider adding elements such as plants, artwork, or a small fountain to enhance the ambiance of the room and create a peaceful environment.

8. Use Props and Accessories: Have props and accessories such as reflexology charts, hand cream, massage oils, and towels readily available for the session. These can enhance the client's experience and make the session more effective.

9. Minimize Distractions: Turn off or silence phones and other electronic devices to minimize distractions during the session. Ensure that the environment is calm and conducive to relaxation.

10. Personalize the Environment: Consider the preferences and needs of the client when setting up the environment. Ask them about their preferences for lighting, music, and scents to create a personalized and comfortable experience.

By setting the right environment for hand reflexology, you can create a peaceful and relaxing space that enhances the effectiveness of the session and promotes overall well-being. Taking the time to create a calming environment can help both you and your client experience the full benefits of hand reflexology.

Techniques for Relaxation in Hand Reflexology

Relaxation is a key component of hand reflexology, as it helps to reduce stress, promote healing, and enhance the overall effectiveness of the session.

Here are some techniques you can use to promote relaxation during a hand reflexology session:

1. Gentle Massage: Begin the session with a gentle hand massage to help relax the muscles and prepare the hands for reflexology. Use long, flowing strokes and gentle kneading motions to help the client unwind.

2. Deep Breathing: Encourage the client to take deep, slow breaths throughout the session. Deep breathing can help to calm the mind and body, reduce stress, and promote relaxation.

3. Progressive Muscle Relaxation: Guide the client through a progressive muscle relaxation exercise, where they tense and then release each muscle group in the body. This can help to release tension and promote relaxation.

4. Visualization: Guide the client through a visualization exercise where they imagine themselves in a peaceful and relaxing place, such as a beach or a forest. Visualization can help to reduce stress and promote a sense of calm.

5. Aromatherapy: Use essential oils or aromatherapy diffusers to infuse the room with relaxing scents. Lavender, chamomile, and sandalwood are known for their calming properties and can help promote relaxation.

6. Soft Music: Play calming music or nature sounds in the background during the session. Soft instrumental music or sounds of nature, such as gentle rain or ocean waves, can help to create a soothing atmosphere.

7. Comfortable Positioning: Ensure that the client is comfortable throughout the session by providing cushions or pillows to support their back and arms. This can help them to relax more fully and enjoy the session.

8. Mindfulness: Encourage the client to practice mindfulness during the session, focusing on the sensations in their hands and letting go of any distracting thoughts. Mindfulness can help to promote relaxation and enhance the benefits of the reflexology session.

9. Warmth: Use warm towels or blankets to keep the client warm and comfortable during the session. Warmth can help to relax the muscles and promote a sense of comfort and well-being.

10. Gentle Touch: Use a gentle and soothing touch during the reflexology session. Avoid using excessive pressure or rough movements, as this can cause discomfort and hinder relaxation.

By incorporating these relaxation techniques into your hand reflexology session, you can help to promote a sense of calm and relaxation for your client. These techniques can enhance the effectiveness of the reflexology session and promote overall well-being.

CHAPTER 5

Mapping the Hand

Detailed Map of the Hands and Corresponding Body Parts

Mapping the hands in reflexology involves identifying specific zones and points that correspond to different parts of the body. While there is no universal standard for mapping the hands, here is a general guide to the reflex points on the hands and their corresponding body parts:

Thumb:

- Tip of the thumb: Head and neck
- Lower thumb: Lungs and respiratory system

- Middle of the thumb: Thyroid gland and endocrine system
- Base of the thumb: Diaphragm and upper abdominal organs

Index Finger:

- Tip of the index finger: Sinuses and frontal area of the head
- Lower index finger: Eyes, ears, and temporal area of the head
- Middle of the index finger: Throat and vocal cords
- Base of the index finger: Digestive system, including stomach and intestines

Middle Finger:

- Tip of the middle finger: Heart and chest area

- Lower middle finger: Liver and gallbladder
- Middle of the middle finger: Circulatory system, including blood vessels and blood pressure
- Base of the middle finger: Adrenal glands and kidneys

Ring Finger:

- Tip of the ring finger: Reproductive organs, including ovaries and testes
- Lower ring finger: Pancreas and insulin production
- Middle of the ring finger: Stomach and spleen
- Base of the ring finger: Urinary system, including bladder and urethra

Little Finger:

- Tip of the little finger: Brain and neurological system

- Lower little finger: Heart and small intestine

- Middle of the little finger: Kidneys and bladder

- Base of the little finger: Pelvic area, including reproductive organs and lower back

Palm:

- Center of the palm: Solar plexus, which is associated with digestion and emotions

- Outer edge of the palm: Spine, with the base of the fingers representing the cervical spine and the wrist representing the lumbar spine

- Base of the fingers: Pelvic area, including reproductive organs and lower back

Mapping the hands in reflexology can help you identify the reflex points that correspond to different parts of the body. By applying pressure to these points, you can help promote healing and relaxation in the corresponding areas, supporting overall health and well-being.

How to Locate Reflex Points on the Hands

Locating reflex points on the hands is a fundamental aspect of hand reflexology.

Here is a step-by-step guide to help you locate reflex points on the hands:

1. Understand the Hand Zones: The hand is divided into zones that correspond to different parts of the body. Each finger represents specific body systems, with the thumb representing the head and neck, the index finger representing the upper body, the middle finger representing the digestive system, the ring finger representing the reproductive system, and the little finger representing the lower body.

2. Use a Reflexology Chart: Refer to a reflexology chart to help you identify the reflex points on the hands. Reflexology charts typically show the location of reflex points on the hands and their corresponding body parts.

3. Start with the Thumb: Begin by locating the reflex points on the thumb. The tip of the thumb corresponds to the head and neck, while the base of the thumb corresponds to the diaphragm and upper abdominal organs.

4. Move to the Fingers: Next, locate the reflex points on the fingers. Each finger corresponds to different body systems, as mentioned earlier. Use your thumb or fingers to apply pressure to these points.

5. Locate the Palm Points: The center of the palm corresponds to the solar plexus, while the outer edge of the palm corresponds to the spine. Use your thumb or fingers to apply pressure to these areas.

6. Use Gentle Pressure: When locating reflex points, use gentle pressure and circular motions to stimulate the points. You should feel a slight tenderness or sensation in the area, which indicates that you have located the reflex point.

7. Be Systematic: Work on one hand at a time, starting with the thumb and moving to the fingers and palm. Be systematic in your approach, ensuring that you cover all the reflex points on the hand.

8. Practice Regularly: With practice, you will become more familiar with the location of reflex points on the hands. Regular practice can help you refine your technique and improve your ability to locate reflex points accurately.

By following these steps, you can effectively locate reflex points on the hands and provide a relaxing and therapeutic hand reflexology session.

Understanding the Connection between Hands and Body in Reflexology

Reflexology is based on the principle that certain areas of the hands (and feet) correspond to specific organs, glands, and other parts of the body. This concept is often referred to as the "reflex arc." The idea is that by applying pressure to these areas, you can stimulate the corresponding body part and promote healing and relaxation.

Here's a deeper look at the connection between the hands and the body in reflexology:

1. Reflex Zones: The hands are divided into reflex zones, each corresponding to different parts of the body. For example, the tips of the fingers correspond to the head and neck, while the base of the fingers corresponds to the lower body.

2. Reflex Points: Within each reflex zone, there are specific reflex points that correspond to specific organs, glands, and body parts. By applying pressure to these points, reflexologists believe they can stimulate the corresponding body part and promote healing.

3. Nerve Pathways: The theory behind reflexology is that there are nerve pathways that connect the reflex points on the hands to the corresponding body parts. By stimulating these nerve pathways, reflexologists believe they can create a response in the corresponding body part.

4. Blood Flow and Energy: Reflexology is also thought to improve blood flow and energy flow throughout the body. By stimulating the reflex points on the hands, reflexologists believe they can improve circulation and energy flow, which can help promote healing and relaxation.

5. Holistic Approach: Reflexology takes a holistic approach to health, treating the whole person rather than just the symptoms of a particular ailment. By addressing imbalances in the body through the hands, reflexologists aim to promote overall health and well-being.

6. Complementary Therapy: Reflexology is often used as a complementary therapy alongside conventional medical treatments. It is not intended to replace medical care but rather to support and enhance it.

Understanding the connection between the hands and the body in reflexology can help you appreciate the principles behind this ancient healing art. By applying pressure to specific points on the hands, reflexologists aim to promote healing, relaxation, and overall well-being in their clients.

CHAPTER 6

Practicing Hand Reflexology

Hand reflexology is a simple yet effective practice that can be done almost anywhere and anytime.

Here are some steps to help you practice hand reflexology:

1. Relaxation: Start by creating a relaxing environment. Sit comfortably in a quiet place where you won't be disturbed. Take a few deep breaths to relax your body and mind.

2. Locate Reflex Points: Use a reflexology chart to locate the reflex points on your hands. These points correspond to different parts of your body. Familiarize yourself with the locations of these points.

3. Apply Pressure: Using your thumb or fingers, apply firm but gentle pressure to the reflex points on your hands. Start with one hand and work your way from the fingers to the palm, covering all the reflex points.

4. Use a Reflexology Tool: You can also use a reflexology tool, such as a hand roller or acupressure ring, to apply pressure to the reflex points. These tools can help you target specific points more effectively.

5. Massage Techniques: Incorporate massage techniques such as kneading, circular motions, and thumb walking to stimulate the reflex points and promote relaxation.

6. Focus on Areas of Discomfort: If you have specific areas of discomfort or tension in your body, focus on the reflex points that correspond to those areas. Apply extra pressure to these points to help relieve tension.

7. Practice Regularly: To experience the full benefits of hand reflexology, practice regularly. Aim for at least 10-15 minutes per hand, several times a week, to promote relaxation and overall well-being.

8. Listen to Your Body: Pay attention to how your body responds to hand reflexology. If you experience any discomfort or pain, stop and consult a healthcare professional.

Practicing hand reflexology can be a soothing and therapeutic practice. By applying pressure to specific points on your hands, you can promote relaxation, relieve tension, and support your overall health and well-being.

Step-by-Step Guide to Performing Hand Reflexology

Performing hand reflexology is a simple and effective way to promote relaxation and support overall health and well-being. **Here is a step-by-step guide to help you perform hand reflexology:**

1. Prepare for the Session:

- Find a quiet and comfortable place to sit.
- Ensure your hands and nails are clean and trimmed.

- Have a reflexology chart and any tools or accessories you may need, such as hand cream or massage oil, ready.

2. Relax and Center Yourself:

- Take a few deep breaths to relax your body and mind.
- Focus on your intention to promote healing and relaxation through hand reflexology.

3. Apply Hand Cream or Massage Oil:

- Apply a small amount of hand cream or massage oil to your hands to lubricate the skin and enhance the reflexology experience.

4. Start with the Thumb:

- Begin by applying gentle pressure to the tip of your thumb with your opposite thumb or index finger. This area corresponds to the head and neck.

5. Move to the Fingers:

- Repeat the process for each finger, working from the tip to the base. Each finger corresponds to different body systems, as mentioned earlier.

6. Massage the Palm:

- Use your thumb or fingers to apply pressure to the reflex points on your palm. Focus on the center of the palm, which corresponds to the solar plexus and digestive system.

7. Use Reflexology Tools (Optional):

- If you have reflexology tools, such as a hand roller or acupressure ring, you can use them to apply pressure to specific points on your hands.

8. Apply Gentle Pressure:

- Use a firm but gentle pressure when applying pressure to the reflex points. You should feel a slight tenderness or sensation in the area, which indicates that you have located the reflex point.

9. Be Systematic:

- Work on one hand at a time, starting with the thumb and moving to the fingers and palm. Be systematic in your approach, ensuring that you cover all the reflex points on the hand.

10. Repeat on the Other Hand:

- Once you have completed the reflexology session on one hand, repeat the process on the other hand to balance the energy flow in your body.

11. Finish with Relaxation Techniques:

- Finish the session by gently massaging your hands and taking a few deep breaths. This can help to integrate the benefits of the reflexology session and promote relaxation.

12. Practice Regularly:

- To experience the full benefits of hand reflexology, practice regularly. Aim for at least 10-15 minutes per hand, several times a week, to promote relaxation and overall well-being.

By following this step-by-step guide, you can effectively perform hand reflexology to promote relaxation, relieve tension, and support your overall health and well-being.

Common Hand Reflexology Techniques

Hand reflexology involves applying pressure to specific points on the hands to stimulate the body's natural healing process.

Here are some common hand reflexology techniques:

1. Thumb Walking: Use your thumb to walk along the reflex points on the hand. Start at the base of the thumb and move towards the tip, applying firm but gentle pressure.

2. Finger Walking: Similar to thumb walking, use your index finger or middle finger to walk along the reflex points on the hand. This technique can be especially effective for smaller reflex points.

3. Rotational Pressing: Apply a circular motion with your thumb or fingers to the reflex points. This technique can help to stimulate the reflex points and promote relaxation.

4. Hook and Back-up: Use your thumb to hook onto a reflex point and then gently back up, applying pressure as you move. This technique can help to release tension in the reflex points.

5. Finger Rolling: Hold the hand in your palm and use your fingers to roll each finger back and forth. This technique can help to stimulate the reflex points on the fingers.

6. Knuckle Technique: Use your knuckles to apply pressure to the reflex points. This technique can be particularly effective for deeper reflex points.

7. Finger Squeezing: Hold the hand in your palm and use your fingers to gently squeeze the reflex points. This can help to stimulate the reflex points and promote relaxation.

8. Wrist Rotation: Hold the wrist with one hand and use the other hand to gently rotate the wrist in a circular motion. This can help to release tension in the wrist and hand.

9. Finger Bending: Hold the hand in your palm and use your fingers to gently bend each finger back and forth. This can help to stimulate the reflex points on the fingers.

10. Thumb Press and Slide: Use your thumb to press firmly on a reflex point and then slide your thumb along the area. This can help to stimulate the reflex points and promote relaxation.

These are just a few of the common hand reflexology techniques that can be used to promote relaxation, relieve tension, and support overall health and well-being. Experiment with these techniques to find what works best for you.

Tips for Effective Hand Reflexology Sessions

Hand reflexology can be a soothing and therapeutic practice when done correctly.

Here are some tips to help you make the most of your hand reflexology sessions:

1. **Prepare the Environment:** Create a quiet and comfortable space for the session. Dim the lights, play soft music, and ensure the temperature is comfortable.

2. **Use Relaxation Techniques:** Start the session with relaxation techniques such as deep breathing or gentle massage to help the client unwind.

3. Focus on the Reflex Points: Use a reflexology chart to locate the reflex points on the hands and focus on applying pressure to these points.

4. Use Proper Technique: Use the appropriate hand reflexology techniques, such as thumb walking or rotational pressing, to stimulate the reflex points effectively.

5. Be Gentle but Firm: Apply gentle but firm pressure to the reflex points. Avoid using excessive force, as this can cause discomfort.

6. Communicate with the Client: Encourage the client to communicate any sensations or feelings they experience during the session. Adjust your pressure or technique based on their feedback.

7. Finish with Relaxation Techniques: End the session with relaxation techniques to help the client transition back to a state of wakefulness.

8. Provide Aftercare Instructions: After the session, provide the client with aftercare instructions, such as drinking plenty of water and practicing self-care techniques at home.

9. Practice Regularly: Regular practice can help you refine your technique and improve your ability to locate reflex points accurately.

10. Seek Professional Training: Consider seeking professional training in hand reflexology to enhance your skills and knowledge.

By following these tips, you can conduct effective hand reflexology sessions that promote relaxation, relieve tension, and support overall health and well-being.

CHAPTER 7

Hand Reflexology for Specific Conditions

Hand reflexology can be used to support the management of various health conditions. While it is not a substitute for medical treatment, it can be a complementary therapy that promotes relaxation and supports overall well-being.

Here are some examples of how hand reflexology can be used for specific conditions:

1. Stress and Anxiety:

- Focus on reflex points that correspond to the adrenal glands, solar plexus, and diaphragm to promote relaxation and reduce stress.

2. Headaches and Migraines:

- Target reflex points on the thumb and fingers that correspond to the head, neck, and sinus areas to help alleviate headache symptoms.

3. Digestive Issues:

- Stimulate reflex points on the fingers and palm that correspond to the digestive organs, such as the stomach and intestines, to support digestion and relieve discomfort.

4. Insomnia:

- Focus on reflex points that correspond to the pituitary gland, pineal gland, and solar plexus to promote relaxation and improve sleep quality.

5. Respiratory Conditions:

- Target reflex points on the thumb and fingers that correspond to the lungs and bronchial tubes to support respiratory function and relieve congestion.

6. Menstrual Cramps:

- Stimulate reflex points on the fingers and palm that correspond to the reproductive organs to help alleviate menstrual cramps and promote hormonal balance.

7. Back Pain:

- Focus on reflex points on the palm and fingers that correspond to the spine and lower back to help relieve tension and discomfort.

8. Fatigue:

- Target reflex points that correspond to the adrenal glands, thyroid gland, and solar plexus to help boost energy levels and reduce fatigue.

9. Arthritis:

- Stimulate reflex points on the fingers and hands that correspond to the joints to help reduce inflammation and improve joint mobility.

10. Circulatory Issues:

- Focus on reflex points that correspond to the circulatory system, such as the heart and blood vessels, to promote healthy circulation and cardiovascular function.

When using hand reflexology for specific conditions, it is important to consult with a healthcare professional to ensure that it is safe and appropriate for your individual needs. Hand reflexology can be a valuable tool for supporting health and well-being, but it should always be used in conjunction with conventional medical treatment when necessary.

Using Hand Reflexology for Pain Relief

Hand reflexology can be an effective natural remedy for managing pain and discomfort in various parts of the body. By stimulating specific reflex points on the hands, you can help alleviate pain and promote relaxation.

Here's how you can use hand reflexology for pain relief:

1. Identify the Reflex Points: Use a reflexology chart to locate the reflex points on the hands that correspond to the area of pain. For example, if you have back pain, focus on the reflex points on the palm and fingers that correspond to the spine and lower back.

2. Apply Pressure: Use your thumb or fingers to apply firm but gentle pressure to the reflex points. Start with a light touch and gradually increase the pressure as tolerated. You should feel a slight tenderness or sensation in the area, which indicates that you have located the reflex point.

3. Use Massage Techniques: Incorporate massage techniques such as kneading, circular motions, and thumb walking to stimulate the reflex points and promote relaxation. Massage can help to increase blood flow and reduce muscle tension, which can help alleviate pain.

4. Focus on Relaxation: As you work on the reflex points, encourage deep breathing and relaxation. This can help to reduce stress and tension, which can contribute to pain.

5. Be Consistent: Practice hand reflexology regularly to experience the full benefits. Aim for at least 10-15 minutes per hand, several times a week, to help manage pain effectively.

6. Consult with a Professional: If you have chronic or severe pain, it's important to consult with a healthcare professional before using hand reflexology as a pain relief method. They can help you determine if hand reflexology is appropriate for your condition and provide guidance on how to use it safely and effectively.

Hand reflexology can be a valuable tool for managing pain and promoting relaxation. By incorporating hand reflexology into your self-care routine, you can help alleviate pain naturally and support your overall health and well-being.

Hand Reflexology for Stress and Anxiety Relief

Hand reflexology can be a soothing and effective way to reduce stress and anxiety. By applying pressure to specific reflex points on the hands, you can help calm the mind and promote relaxation.

Here's how you can use hand reflexology for stress and anxiety relief:

1. Relaxation Techniques: Start by creating a calming environment. Sit in a comfortable position and take a few deep breaths to relax your body and mind.

2. Locate the Reflex Points: Use a reflexology chart to locate the reflex points on your hands that correspond to stress and anxiety relief. These points are typically located on the thumb, fingers, and palm.

3. Apply Pressure: Use your thumb or fingers to apply firm but gentle pressure to the reflex points. Start with the reflex points on one hand and then move to the other hand.

4. Massage Techniques: Use massage techniques such as kneading, circular motions, and thumb walking to stimulate the reflex points and promote relaxation. Focus on applying pressure to the reflex points that correspond to the adrenal glands, solar plexus, and diaphragm.

5. Deep Breathing: Encourage deep breathing as you work on the reflex points. Deep breathing can help to further relax the body and mind, reducing stress and anxiety.

6. Be Consistent: Practice hand reflexology regularly to experience the full benefits. Aim for at least 10-15 minutes per hand, several times a week, to help manage stress and anxiety effectively.

7. Consult with a Professional: If you have severe or chronic stress and anxiety, it's important to consult with a healthcare professional. They can help you determine if hand reflexology is appropriate for your condition and provide guidance on how to use it safely and effectively.

Hand reflexology can be a valuable tool for reducing stress and anxiety. By incorporating hand reflexology into your self-care routine, you can help calm your mind, relax your body, and promote overall well-being.

Hand Reflexology for Better Sleep

Hand reflexology can be a helpful natural remedy for improving sleep quality. By stimulating specific reflex points on the hands, you can help calm the mind and promote relaxation, which can lead to better sleep.

Here's how you can use hand reflexology for better sleep:

1. Relaxation Techniques: Start by creating a calming environment. Sit in a comfortable position and take a few deep breaths to relax your body and mind.

2. Locate the Reflex Points: Use a reflexology chart to locate the reflex points on your hands that correspond to sleep and relaxation. These points are typically located on the fingers and palm.

3. Apply Pressure: Use your thumb or fingers to apply firm but gentle pressure to the reflex points. Start with the reflex points on one hand and then move to the other hand.

4. Massage Techniques: Use massage techniques such as kneading, circular motions, and thumb walking to stimulate the reflex points and promote relaxation. Focus on applying pressure to the reflex points that correspond to the pituitary gland, pineal gland, and solar plexus.

5. Deep Breathing: Encourage deep breathing as you work on the reflex points. Deep breathing can help to further relax the body and promote better sleep.

6. Be Consistent: Practice hand reflexology regularly to experience the full benefits. Aim for at least 10-15 minutes per hand, several times a week, to help improve sleep quality.

7. Create a Bedtime Routine: Incorporate hand reflexology into your bedtime routine to help signal to your body that it's time to wind down and prepare for sleep.

8. Consult with a Professional: If you have chronic sleep issues, it's important to consult with a healthcare professional. They can help you determine if hand reflexology is appropriate for your condition and provide guidance on how to use it safely and effectively.

Hand reflexology can be a valuable tool for promoting relaxation and improving sleep quality. By incorporating hand reflexology into your self-care routine, you can help support better sleep and overall well-being.

CHAPTER 8

Incorporating Hand Reflexology Into Your Wellness Routine

Hand reflexology can be a valuable addition to your wellness routine, helping to promote relaxation, reduce stress, and support overall health and well-being.

Here are some tips for incorporating hand reflexology into your wellness routine:

1. Schedule Regular Sessions: Set aside time each day or week for hand reflexology sessions. Even just 10-15 minutes can be beneficial.

2. Create a Relaxing Environment: Find a quiet and comfortable space for your hand reflexology sessions. Dim the lights, play calming music, and create a soothing atmosphere.

3. Use Essential Oils: Consider using essential oils known for their relaxing properties, such as lavender or chamomile, during your hand reflexology sessions.

4. Practice Deep Breathing: Incorporate deep breathing exercises into your hand reflexology sessions to enhance relaxation.

5. Combine with Other Relaxation Techniques: Consider combining hand reflexology with other relaxation techniques, such as meditation or yoga, for a more comprehensive wellness routine.

6. Stay Consistent: Make hand reflexology a regular part of your wellness routine to experience the full benefits.

7. Listen to Your Body: Pay attention to how your body responds to hand reflexology. Adjust your technique or pressure based on what feels comfortable and effective for you.

8. Seek Professional Training: Consider seeking professional training in hand reflexology to enhance your skills and knowledge.

9. Be Mindful of Your Hands: Throughout the day, be mindful of your hands and how you use them. Avoid excessive strain or tension, and practice gentle stretching exercises to keep your hands flexible and relaxed.

10. Consult with a Professional: If you have specific health concerns or conditions, consult with a healthcare professional before incorporating hand reflexology into your wellness routine.

By incorporating hand reflexology into your wellness routine, you can help promote relaxation, reduce stress, and support your overall health and well-being. Experiment with different techniques and find what works best for you.

Integrating Hand Reflexology with Other Wellness Practices

Integrating hand reflexology with other wellness practices can enhance its benefits and promote overall well-being.

Here are some ways to integrate hand reflexology with other wellness practices:

1. Massage Therapy: Combine hand reflexology with full-body massage therapy to promote relaxation and relieve tension throughout the body.

2. Aromatherapy: Use essential oils during hand reflexology sessions to enhance relaxation and promote a sense of well-being. Lavender, chamomile, and frankincense are popular choices for relaxation.

3. Meditation: Practice mindfulness meditation before or after hand reflexology sessions to calm the mind and enhance relaxation.

4. Yoga: Incorporate hand reflexology into your yoga practice by massaging your hands before or after yoga poses to release tension and promote relaxation.

5. Breathing Exercises: Combine hand reflexology with deep breathing exercises to enhance relaxation and reduce stress.

6. Acupressure: Use acupressure techniques on the hands along with hand reflexology to stimulate energy flow and promote overall well-being.

7. Stretching: Practice gentle hand and wrist stretches to complement hand reflexology and promote flexibility and relaxation in the hands.

8. Mindful Movement: Engage in mindful movement practices such as tai chi or qigong to complement hand reflexology and promote overall relaxation and well-being.

9. Healthy Diet: Maintain a healthy diet rich in fruits, vegetables, whole grains, and lean proteins to support overall health and well-being, including the health of your hands.

10. Hydration: Stay hydrated by drinking plenty of water throughout the day to support overall health and well-being, including the health of your hands.

Integrating hand reflexology with other wellness practices can enhance its benefits and promote overall well-being. Experiment with different combinations to find what works best for you.

Daily Hand Reflexology Exercises for Self-Care

Incorporating hand reflexology into your daily routine can be a simple yet effective way to promote relaxation, reduce stress, and support overall well-being.

Here are some daily hand reflexology exercises you can practice for self-care:

1. Morning Wake-Up: Start your day with a quick hand reflexology session to help wake up your body and mind. Focus on stimulating reflex points that correspond to energy and vitality, such as the adrenal glands and solar plexus.

2. Midday Relaxation: Take a break during the day to practice hand reflexology and relax your mind and body. Focus on reflex points that correspond to stress relief, such as the diaphragm and pituitary gland.

3. Evening Wind-Down: Wind down in the evening with a calming hand reflexology session to prepare your body for restful sleep. Focus on reflex points that correspond to relaxation and sleep, such as the pineal gland and solar plexus.

4. Stress Relief: Whenever you feel stressed or tense, take a few minutes to practice hand reflexology. Focus on reflex points that correspond to stress relief, such as the adrenal glands and diaphragm.

5. Digestive Support: If you experience digestive discomfort, practice hand reflexology to support digestion. Focus on reflex points that correspond to the digestive organs, such as the stomach and intestines.

6. Energy Boost: When you need a quick energy boost, practice hand reflexology to stimulate energy flow. Focus on reflex points that correspond to energy and vitality, such as the adrenal glands and solar plexus.

7. Overall Well-Being: Incorporate hand reflexology into your daily routine as part of your overall self-care practice. Focus on stimulating reflex points that correspond to various organs and systems of the body to promote overall health and well-being.

By incorporating these daily hand reflexology exercises into your routine, you can help promote relaxation, reduce stress, and support your overall health and well-being. Adjust the exercises to suit your needs and preferences, and enjoy the benefits of this simple yet powerful self-care practice.

Maintaining Hand Health for Reflexology

Maintaining the health of your hands is essential for practicing hand reflexology effectively.

Here are some tips to help you keep your hands healthy and in optimal condition for reflexology:

1. Regular Stretching: Incorporate hand and wrist stretching exercises into your daily routine to keep your hands flexible and prevent stiffness.

2. Proper Posture: Maintain good posture during reflexology sessions to reduce strain on your hands and wrists. Sit up straight and avoid hunching over.

3. Hand Care: Keep your hands clean and moisturized to prevent dryness and cracking. Use a gentle hand cream regularly to keep your skin hydrated.

4. Nail Care: Keep your nails trimmed and clean to prevent them from scratching or causing discomfort during reflexology sessions.

5. Use Proper Technique: Use proper hand reflexology techniques to avoid unnecessary strain on your hands and wrists. Apply pressure using your thumb or fingers in a gentle but firm manner.

6. Rest and Recovery: Give your hands time to rest and recover after reflexology sessions. Avoid overworking your hands and take breaks when needed.

7. Use Tools: Consider using reflexology tools such as hand rollers or acupressure rings to reduce strain on your hands and fingers.

8. Stay Hydrated: Drink plenty of water to keep your body and hands hydrated, which can help prevent cramping and stiffness.

9. Exercise Regularly: Engage in regular physical activity to maintain overall hand and wrist strength and flexibility.

10. Seek Professional Help: If you experience persistent pain or discomfort in your hands, seek the advice of a healthcare professional. They can help you determine the cause of your symptoms and recommend appropriate treatment.

By following these tips, you can help maintain the health of your hands and wrists for practicing hand reflexology effectively. Prioritize self-care and hand health to ensure that you can continue to enjoy the benefits of reflexology for years to come.

CHAPTER 9

Advanced Hand Reflexology Techniques

For those looking to deepen their understanding and practice of hand reflexology, advanced techniques can provide additional benefits and therapeutic effects.

Here are some advanced hand reflexology techniques to consider:

1. Zone Therapy: This technique involves dividing the hands into zones that correspond to different areas of the body. By applying pressure to specific zones, you can target corresponding organs and systems.

2. Meridian Reflexology: Similar to acupuncture meridians, this technique involves stimulating meridian points on the hands to promote energy flow and balance in the body.

3. Chakra Reflexology: Chakras are energy centers in the body. This technique involves stimulating reflex points on the hands that correspond to the chakras to promote balance and alignment.

4. Lymphatic Drainage: By using gentle, rhythmic movements on the hands, you can stimulate the lymphatic system and promote the removal of toxins and waste from the body.

5. Joint Mobilization: This technique involves gently mobilizing the joints of the fingers and hands to improve flexibility and range of motion.

6. Craniosacral Reflexology: This technique focuses on reflex points on the hands that correspond to the craniosacral system, which includes the skull, spine, and sacrum. It aims to promote relaxation and balance in this system.

7. Trigger Point Therapy: By identifying and applying pressure to trigger points in the hands, you can help relieve tension and pain in corresponding areas of the body.

8. Combination Techniques: Advanced practitioners often combine different hand reflexology techniques to create a customized treatment plan for their clients, based on their individual needs and goals.

9.   Emotional   Release: Some   advanced techniques   focus   on   reflex   points   that   are believed   to   be   connected   to   emotions.   By stimulating   these   points,   practitioners   aim   to release emotional tension and promote emotional well-being.

10.   Self-Reflexology   Techniques: Advanced practitioners   may   also   teach   clients self-reflexology techniques that they can practice at   home   to   enhance   the   effects   of   professional treatments.

These   advanced   hand   reflexology   techniques require additional training and practice to master. If you're interested in learning more about these techniques,   consider   seeking   out   a   qualified reflexology   practitioner   or   attending   advanced training courses.

Advanced Hand Reflexology Points and Zones

In advanced hand reflexology, practitioners focus on specific points and zones on the hands that correspond to different organs, systems, and areas of the body.

Here are some advanced hand reflexology points and zones to consider:

1. Thumb:

- Corresponds to the head and neck area.
- Stimulating this point can help alleviate headaches and neck tension.

2. Index Finger:

- Corresponds to the sinuses and respiratory system.

- Stimulating this point can help relieve sinus congestion and respiratory issues.

3. Middle Finger:

- Corresponds to the digestive system.
- Stimulating this point can help improve digestion and relieve digestive discomfort.

4. Ring Finger:

- Corresponds to the reproductive system.
- Stimulating this point can help balance hormonal levels and support reproductive health.

5. Little Finger:

- Corresponds to the heart and small intestine.

- Stimulating this point can help support heart health and improve digestion.

6. Palm:

- Divided into zones that correspond to different parts of the body.
- Zone 1: Corresponds to the chest and upper back.
- Zone 2: Corresponds to the stomach and lower back.
- Zone 3: Corresponds to the pelvis and lower body.

7. Back of Hand:

- Also divided into zones that correspond to different parts of the body.
- Zone 4: Corresponds to the head and neck.

- Zone 5: Corresponds to the upper back and chest.
- Zone 6: Corresponds to the lower back and pelvis.

8. Wrist:

- Corresponds to the ankles and feet.
- Stimulating this area can help relieve foot and ankle pain.

By focusing on these advanced hand reflexology points and zones, practitioners can provide targeted treatment to address specific health issues and promote overall well-being. It's important to receive training from a qualified reflexology practitioner before attempting advanced hand reflexology techniques.

Reflexology for Emotional Wellbeing through the Hands

Reflexology can be a powerful tool for promoting emotional well-being by stimulating specific reflex points on the hands that are believed to be connected to emotions.

Here are some ways in which hand reflexology can support emotional health:

1. Stress Relief: By stimulating reflex points on the hands that correspond to the adrenal glands and solar plexus, hand reflexology can help reduce stress and promote relaxation.

2. Anxiety Reduction: Reflexology can help reduce anxiety by focusing on reflex points that correspond to the diaphragm and pituitary gland, which are associated with relaxation and calming effects.

3. Mood Enhancement: By targeting reflex points that correspond to the brain and nervous system, hand reflexology can help enhance mood and promote a sense of well-being.

4. Emotional Release: Reflexology can stimulate reflex points that are believed to be connected to emotions, helping to release emotional tension and promote emotional balance.

5. Relaxation Response: Hand reflexology can trigger the body's relaxation response, which can help reduce feelings of stress and anxiety.

6. Self-Care Practice: Practicing hand reflexology on yourself can be a form of self-care, providing a calming and nurturing experience that supports emotional well-being.

7. Holistic Approach: Reflexology takes a holistic approach to health, treating the whole person and addressing emotional, mental, and physical aspects of well-being.

8. Support for Mental Health: Reflexology can be a complementary therapy for supporting mental health conditions such as depression and anxiety, promoting relaxation and reducing symptoms.

9. Mind-Body Connection: Reflexology recognizes the connection between the mind and body, and by working on the hands, it can help balance emotions and promote overall well-being.

10. Stress Management: Reflexology can be used as a tool for managing stress, providing a natural and non-invasive way to promote relaxation and emotional balance.

Overall, hand reflexology can be a gentle yet effective way to support emotional well-being, providing relaxation, stress relief, and emotional balance. It can be used as part of a holistic approach to health and well-being, promoting overall emotional health and wellness.

Hand Reflexology for Energy Balance

Hand reflexology is believed to help balance the body's energy by stimulating specific reflex points on the hands that correspond to different organs and systems.

Here's how hand reflexology can promote energy balance:

1. Stimulating Energy Flow: By applying pressure to reflex points on the hands, hand reflexology is thought to stimulate the flow of energy, or "qi," through the body's meridians, promoting balance and vitality.

2. Clearing Blockages: It is believed that hand reflexology can help clear blockages in the body's energy pathways, allowing energy to flow freely and restoring balance.

3. Balancing Chakras: Hand reflexology can be used to balance the body's chakras, or energy centers, by stimulating reflex points on the hands that correspond to each chakra.

4. Enhancing Vitality: By promoting energy balance, hand reflexology can help enhance overall vitality and well-being.

5. Stress Reduction: Hand reflexology can help reduce stress, which can disrupt the body's energy flow and lead to imbalances.

6. Emotional Balance: Hand reflexology can support emotional balance by helping to release emotional tension and promote relaxation, which can contribute to overall energy balance.

7. Supporting the Body's Natural Healing Process: By promoting energy balance, hand reflexology can support the body's natural healing process, allowing it to function optimally.

8. Enhancing Well-Being: Hand reflexology is believed to enhance overall well-being by promoting energy balance and vitality.

9. Self-Care Practice: Practicing hand reflexology on yourself can be a form of self-care that supports energy balance and overall well-being.

10. Holistic Approach: Hand reflexology takes a holistic approach to health, addressing the physical, emotional, and energetic aspects of well-being to promote overall balance and vitality.

Overall, hand reflexology can be a gentle yet effective way to promote energy balance and enhance overall well-being. It can be used as part of a holistic approach to health, supporting the body's natural ability to heal and maintain balance.

CHAPTER 10

Exploring Reflexology Traditions

Reflexology is a practice that has roots in various cultures and traditions around the world. **Here are some of the key traditions and their approaches to reflexology:**

1. Traditional Chinese Medicine (TCM): In TCM, reflexology is based on the principles of meridians, or energy pathways, that run throughout the body. By stimulating specific points on the hands, feet, and ears, practitioners aim to restore balance and harmony to the body's energy flow.

2. Ayurveda: In Ayurvedic medicine, reflexology is known as "marma therapy" and is based on the concept of vital energy, or "prana," flowing through the body. By stimulating specific points on the hands and feet, practitioners aim to balance the doshas (vata, pitta, and kapha) and promote overall health and well-being.

3. Ancient Egypt: The ancient Egyptians practiced reflexology as early as 2500-2330 BCE, as evidenced by a pictograph depicting reflexology points on the feet found in the physician's tomb in Saqqara. They believed that the feet were a map of the body and that applying pressure to specific points could promote healing.

4. Native American Traditions: Some Native American tribes, such as the Cherokee, practiced a form of reflexology known as "foot walking," where practitioners would walk on the recipient's back and feet to stimulate healing and balance energy flow.

5. European Traditions: In Europe, reflexology has roots in traditional healing practices dating back to ancient Greece and Rome. In the Middle Ages, European monks practiced a form of foot reflexology as part of their healing traditions.

6. Modern Reflexology: Modern reflexology as we know it today was developed in the early 20th century by Eunice Ingham, a physiotherapist who mapped the reflex points on the feet and hands and developed techniques for stimulating them. Her work laid the foundation for the modern practice of reflexology.

7. Global Influence: Reflexology has been influenced by various cultures and traditions around the world, including Traditional Chinese Medicine, Ayurveda, and Native American healing practices. Today, reflexology is practiced worldwide and continues to evolve as a holistic healing modality.

Overall, reflexology is a practice that has deep roots in various cultures and traditions, each with its own unique approach to healing and well-being. By exploring these traditions, we can gain a deeper understanding of the principles and practices that underpin reflexology and its role in promoting health and wellness.

Different Traditions and Approaches to Hand Reflexology

Hand reflexology is a practice that has been adapted and incorporated into various healing traditions around the world.

Here are some of the different traditions and approaches to hand reflexology:

1. Traditional Chinese Medicine (TCM): In TCM, hand reflexology is based on the principles of meridians, or energy pathways, that run throughout the body. By stimulating specific points on the hands, practitioners aim to restore balance and harmony to the body's energy flow.

2. Ayurveda: In Ayurvedic medicine, hand reflexology is known as "hasta marma" and is based on the concept of vital energy, or "prana," flowing through the body. By stimulating specific points on the hands, practitioners aim to balance the doshas (vata, pitta, and kapha) and promote overall health and well-being.

3. Native American Traditions: Some Native American tribes incorporate hand reflexology into their healing practices, using it as a way to stimulate energy flow and promote balance in the body.

4. European Traditions: In Europe, hand reflexology has been practiced for centuries as part of traditional healing practices. It was often used in conjunction with other therapies to promote health and well-being.

5. Modern Reflexology: Modern hand reflexology is based on the work of Eunice

Ingham, who mapped the reflex points on the hands and developed techniques for stimulating them. Her work laid the foundation for the modern practice of hand reflexology, which is used worldwide today.

6. Integrative Approaches: In recent years, hand reflexology has been integrated into various holistic and integrative approaches to health and wellness. It is often used in conjunction with other therapies such as massage, acupuncture, and aromatherapy to promote overall well-being.

Overall, hand reflexology is a versatile and effective healing modality that has been adapted and incorporated into various healing traditions around the world. Whether used as a standalone therapy or as part of a larger treatment plan, hand reflexology can help promote balance, relaxation, and overall health and well-being.

Cultural and Historical Perspectives on Hand Reflexology

Hand reflexology has a rich history that spans across various cultures and traditions.

Here are some cultural and historical perspectives on hand reflexology:

1. Ancient Egypt: The ancient Egyptians are believed to have practiced reflexology as early as 2500-2330 BCE. Evidence of this can be seen in a pictograph found in the physician's tomb in Saqqara, which depicts reflexology points on the feet. The Egyptians believed that the feet were a map of the body and that applying pressure to specific points could promote healing.

2. Traditional Chinese Medicine (TCM): Hand reflexology is rooted in TCM, which dates back thousands of years. In TCM, it is believed that the hands contain reflex points that correspond to different organs and systems in the body. By stimulating these points, practitioners aim to restore balance and harmony to the body's energy flow.

3. Ayurveda: In Ayurvedic medicine, hand reflexology is known as "hasta marma" and is based on the concept of vital energy, or "prana," flowing through the body. By stimulating specific points on the hands, practitioners aim to balance the doshas (vata, pitta, and kapha) and promote overall health and well-being.

4. Native American Traditions: Some Native American tribes incorporate hand reflexology into their healing practices, using it as a way to stimulate energy flow and promote balance in the body. Hand reflexology is often used in conjunction with other traditional healing modalities, such as herbal medicine and energy work.

5. European Traditions: Hand reflexology has been practiced in Europe for centuries as part of traditional healing practices. It was often used in conjunction with other therapies to promote health and well-being. In the Middle Ages, European monks practiced a form of foot reflexology as part of their healing traditions.

6. Modern Reflexology: Modern hand reflexology as we know it today was developed in the early 20th century by Eunice Ingham, a physiotherapist who mapped the reflex points on the hands and developed techniques for stimulating them. Her work laid the foundation for the modern practice of hand reflexology, which is used worldwide today.

Overall, hand reflexology has a long and diverse history, with roots in various cultures and traditions around the world. Whether used for healing, relaxation, or overall well-being, hand reflexology continues to be a valuable practice that has stood the test of time.

Modern Innovations in Hand Reflexology

While hand reflexology has deep roots in ancient traditions, modern innovations have expanded its practice and effectiveness.

Here are some modern innovations in hand reflexology:

1. **Reflexology Tools:** Various tools, such as hand rollers, balls, and sticks, have been developed to enhance the effectiveness of hand reflexology. These tools can help apply pressure to specific reflex points more effectively and can be used for self-care between professional sessions.

2. **Technology:** Some practitioners use technology, such as reflexology gloves or socks

with embedded sensors, to provide feedback on pressure and technique. This can help ensure that the correct reflex points are being targeted and that the right amount of pressure is being applied.

3. Virtual Sessions: With the rise of telehealth and virtual consultations, some reflexologists offer virtual hand reflexology sessions. These sessions allow clients to receive personalized instruction and guidance on hand reflexology techniques from the comfort of their own home.

4. Integrative Approaches: Many modern reflexologists integrate other modalities into their practice, such as aromatherapy, massage, and acupressure. These integrative approaches can enhance the overall effectiveness of hand reflexology and provide a more holistic healing experience.

5. Research and Evidence-Based Practice: Modern research has helped validate the effectiveness of hand reflexology for various health conditions. Reflexologists now use evidence-based practices to tailor treatments to individual needs and ensure the best possible outcomes.

6. Specialized Techniques: Some practitioners have developed specialized techniques for hand reflexology, such as zone therapy and craniosacral reflexology. These techniques target specific reflex points on the hands to address specific health issues or promote overall well-being.

7. Continuing Education: Reflexologists now have access to a wide range of continuing education opportunities to expand their knowledge and skills. This allows them to stay up-to-date with the latest research and techniques in hand reflexology.

Overall, modern innovations in hand reflexology have helped expand its practice and effectiveness, making it a valuable tool for promoting health and well-being in today's world.

CHAPTER 11

Frequently Asked Questions about Hand Reflexology

1. What is hand reflexology?

- Hand reflexology is a holistic healing technique that involves applying pressure to specific points on the hands to promote relaxation, reduce stress, and stimulate healing in other parts of the body.

2. How does hand reflexology work?

- Hand reflexology is based on the principle that there are reflex points on the hands that correspond to different organs, glands, and parts of the body. By stimulating these points, practitioners believe they can promote balance and harmony in the body's energy flow.

3. What are the benefits of hand reflexology?

- Hand reflexology can help reduce stress, promote relaxation, improve circulation, enhance overall well-being, and support the body's natural healing process.

4. Is hand reflexology painful?

- Hand reflexology should not be painful. The pressure applied should be firm but gentle. If you experience any discomfort during a session, be sure to communicate with your reflexologist so they can adjust the pressure accordingly.

5. How long does a hand reflexology session last?

- A typical hand reflexology session lasts between 30 to 60 minutes. However, shorter or longer sessions can also be beneficial depending on your needs and preferences.

6. How often should I receive hand reflexology treatments?

- The frequency of hand reflexology treatments can vary depending on your individual needs and goals. Some people benefit from weekly sessions, while others may find monthly sessions sufficient. It's best to discuss a treatment plan with your reflexologist based on your specific needs.

7. Can I perform hand reflexology on myself?

- Yes, hand reflexology can be performed on yourself. There are many resources available, such as books, videos, and online tutorials, that can guide you through the process. However, for best results, it's recommended to receive treatment from a trained reflexologist.

8. Is hand reflexology safe for everyone?

- Hand reflexology is generally safe for most people. However, if you have a serious medical condition or are pregnant, it's important to consult with your healthcare provider before starting any new treatment, including hand reflexology.

9. How can I find a qualified hand reflexologist?

- To find a qualified hand reflexologist, you can ask for recommendations from friends or family, search online directories, or contact professional reflexology associations for referrals.

10. Can hand reflexology help with specific health conditions?

- While hand reflexology is not a substitute for medical treatment, it can be used as a complementary therapy to support overall health and well-being. Some people find relief from conditions such as headaches, digestive issues, and chronic pain through hand reflexology. It's best to consult with a qualified reflexologist to discuss your specific health concerns.

Addressing Common Concerns and Misconceptions about Hand Reflexology

Hand reflexology is a widely practiced holistic therapy that offers numerous benefits. However, there are some common concerns and misconceptions that people may have.

Here, I address these concerns and provide clarity on some misconceptions:

1. Concern: Reflexology is painful.

Clarification: Reflexology, including hand reflexology, should not be painful. The pressure applied should be firm but gentle, and you should communicate with your reflexologist if you experience any discomfort.

2. Concern: Reflexology is only for relaxation.

Clarification: While reflexology is indeed relaxing, it offers a range of benefits beyond relaxation. It can help improve circulation, reduce stress, and support overall health and well-being.

3. Concern: Reflexology is not based on scientific evidence.

Clarification: While more research is needed, there is evidence to support the effectiveness of reflexology for various health conditions. Many people find it to be a valuable complement to conventional medical treatments.

4. Concern: Reflexology is only for feet.

Clarification: While foot reflexology is more well-known, hand reflexology is also a popular and effective form of reflexology. Both modalities work on the same principle of stimulating reflex points to promote healing and balance in the body.

5. Concern: Reflexology can cure diseases.
Clarification: Reflexology is not a cure for diseases. It is a complementary therapy that can help support the body's natural healing process and promote overall health and well-being.

6. Concern: Reflexology is not safe for pregnant women.
Clarification: Reflexology can be safe for pregnant women when performed by a qualified reflexologist who is experienced in working with pregnant clients. It can help promote relaxation and alleviate pregnancy-related discomforts.

7. Concern: Reflexology is only for adults.

Clarification: Reflexology can be beneficial for people of all ages, including children and the elderly. However, the pressure and techniques used may be adjusted depending on the individual's age and health condition.

8. Concern: Reflexology is a luxury treatment. Clarification: While reflexology can be a relaxing and enjoyable experience, it is also a therapeutic treatment that offers numerous health benefits. Many people incorporate reflexology into their wellness routine for its holistic benefits.

By addressing these common concerns and misconceptions, we hope to provide a clearer understanding of the benefits and safety of hand reflexology as a holistic therapy.

Tips for Enhancing Your Hand Reflexology Practice

Whether you're a seasoned reflexologist or just starting out, there are several tips you can use to enhance your hand reflexology practice. **Here are some suggestions:**

1. Continuing Education: Stay updated with the latest research and techniques in hand reflexology by attending workshops, seminars, and conferences. Continuing education can help you expand your knowledge and skills.

2. Practice Self-Reflexology: Regularly practice hand reflexology on yourself to maintain your skills and experience the benefits firsthand. Self-reflexology can also help you understand the technique from the client's perspective.

3. Keep Your Hands Healthy: Maintain good hand hygiene and take care of your hands to ensure they are in optimal condition for performing reflexology. Consider using hand creams or oils to keep your hands soft and supple.

4. Use Props and Tools: Experiment with different props and tools, such as reflexology gloves, balls, or rollers, to enhance your practice. These tools can help you apply pressure more effectively and provide a different sensory experience for your clients.

5. Customize Your Approach: Tailor your hand reflexology sessions to meet the individual needs of your clients. Pay attention to their feedback and adjust your techniques accordingly to provide a personalized experience.

6. Combine Modalities: Consider integrating other holistic modalities, such as aromatherapy, acupressure, or Reiki, into your hand reflexology sessions to enhance the overall experience for your clients.

7. Maintain Professionalism: Create a relaxing and professional environment for your clients by ensuring your workspace is clean, comfortable, and free from distractions. Professionalism helps build trust and credibility with your clients.

8. Stay Connected: Network with other reflexologists and healthcare professionals to stay connected with the broader holistic health community. Collaboration and knowledge-sharing can help you grow as a practitioner.

9. Seek Feedback: Encourage feedback from your clients to help you improve your practice. Listen to their suggestions and incorporate them into your sessions where appropriate.

10. Stay Passionate: Lastly, stay passionate and curious about hand reflexology. Continuously seek to deepen your understanding and appreciation for this ancient healing art.

By incorporating these tips into your hand reflexology practice, you can enhance the effectiveness of your sessions and provide a more holistic and rewarding experience for your clients.

Troubleshooting Issues during Hand Reflexology Sessions

Hand reflexology sessions can sometimes present challenges or issues that require troubleshooting.

Here are some common issues and tips on how to address them:

1. Client Discomfort: If your client experiences discomfort during the session, adjust your pressure and technique. Use a lighter touch or focus on other areas of the hand. Communication is key—ask for feedback and adjust accordingly.

2. Lack of Response: If your client does not seem to be responding to the reflexology treatment, try changing your approach. Use different techniques or focus on different reflex points. It's also possible that the client may need more sessions to experience the full benefits.

3. Hand Sensitivity: Some clients may have sensitive hands, making the reflexology session uncomfortable. Use a gentler touch and adjust your pressure accordingly. You can also use props or tools to apply pressure more evenly and gently.

4. Fatigue: Reflexology can be physically demanding, especially if you are performing multiple sessions in a day. Take breaks between sessions to rest and recharge. Practice self-care techniques, such as hand stretches, to prevent fatigue and strain.

5. Client Expectations: Sometimes, clients may have unrealistic expectations about the benefits of reflexology. Manage expectations by explaining the purpose and limitations of reflexology. Encourage clients to approach reflexology as a complementary therapy rather than a cure-all.

6. Emotional Release: Reflexology can sometimes trigger emotional release in clients, leading to unexpected emotions or reactions. Provide a supportive environment for clients to process their emotions and assure them that it is a normal part of the healing process.

7. Inconsistent Results: If you are not seeing consistent results with your clients, revisit your technique and approach. Consider seeking feedback from colleagues or attending additional training to improve your skills.

8. Client Communication: Effective communication is key to a successful reflexology session. Listen to your client's feedback and adjust your approach accordingly. Encourage open and honest communication to ensure a positive experience for both you and your client.

By addressing these common issues and implementing the suggested tips, you can troubleshoot challenges that may arise during hand reflexology sessions and ensure a more effective and enjoyable experience for your clients.

CHAPTER 12

The Future of Hand Reflexology

Hand reflexology has a long history and a promising future as a holistic therapy.

Here are some potential developments and trends that could shape the future of hand reflexology:

1. Integration with Technology: As technology advances, we may see the integration of hand reflexology with digital tools and devices. This could include the development of apps or wearable devices that provide guided hand reflexology sessions or track reflexology points and pressure.

2. Research and Evidence-Based Practice: Continued research into the effectiveness of hand reflexology for various health conditions could help solidify its place in mainstream healthcare. More studies may lead to increased acceptance and integration of hand reflexology into conventional medical settings.

3. Specialized Training and Certification: As interest in hand reflexology grows, we may see more specialized training programs and certification options for reflexologists. This could help ensure that practitioners are well-trained and skilled in providing effective hand reflexology treatments.

4. Personalized Treatment Plans: With a greater understanding of individual differences, hand reflexology treatments may become more personalized. Reflexologists may tailor treatments based on a client's specific needs, health goals, and even genetic makeup.

5. Integration with Other Holistic Modalities: Hand reflexology may be increasingly integrated with other holistic modalities, such as aromatherapy, acupuncture, or yoga. This integrated approach could provide more comprehensive and effective care for clients.

6. Increased Accessibility: Advances in technology and training may make hand reflexology more accessible to a wider range of people. This could include virtual sessions, self-care resources, and community outreach programs.

7. Recognition and Regulation: As hand reflexology gains popularity, there may be increased recognition and regulation of the practice. This could include standardized training requirements, licensing, and professional standards to ensure quality and safety.

8. Collaboration with Conventional Medicine: Hand reflexology may become more integrated into conventional healthcare settings, with practitioners collaborating with medical professionals to provide complementary care for patients.

Overall, the future of hand reflexology looks promising, with potential developments that could enhance its effectiveness, accessibility, and integration into mainstream healthcare. As research and practice continue to evolve, hand reflexology has the potential to play an increasingly important role in promoting health and well-being.

Final Thoughts and Encouragement for Practitioners of Hand Reflexology

As a practitioner of hand reflexology, you have chosen a path that offers immense potential for healing and well-being. Your dedication to this ancient healing art is commendable, and your commitment to helping others is truly inspiring. **Here are some final thoughts and encouragement for you:**

1. Believe in the Power of Hand Reflexology: Hand reflexology has a long history of promoting health and well-being. Trust in the power of this practice to support your clients' healing journeys.

2. Continue Learning and Growing: Stay curious and open to new knowledge and techniques. Continued learning will not only benefit your clients but also enrich your own practice.

3. Listen to Your Clients: Your clients' feedback is invaluable. Listen attentively to their needs and concerns, and tailor your treatments accordingly.

4. Take Care of Yourself: Practicing self-care is essential for maintaining your own health and well-being. Remember to rest, recharge, and seek support when needed.

5. Be Patient and Persistent: Building a successful reflexology practice takes time and effort. Stay patient and persistent, and trust that your dedication will pay off.

6. Celebrate Your Successes: Take time to celebrate your successes, no matter how small. Each client you help is a testament to the impact of your work.

7. Stay Connected: Connect with other reflexology practitioners and holistic health professionals. Share your experiences, learn from others, and stay inspired.

8. Trust Your Intuition: As a reflexologist, you have a unique intuition that guides your practice.

Trust in your instincts and let them guide you in your treatments.

9. Be Grateful: Be grateful for the opportunity to practice hand reflexology and make a positive difference in the lives of others. Your work is meaningful and appreciated.

10. Keep the Passion Alive: Finally, keep the passion for hand reflexology alive in your heart. Your passion is what drives you to excel in your practice and make a difference in the world.

Thank you for your dedication to the art of hand reflexology. Your work is truly valuable, and you have the potential to touch many lives with your healing touch.

CHAPTER 13

Key Terms and Concepts in Hand Reflexology

1. Reflexology: A holistic therapy based on the principle that there are reflex points on the hands (and feet) that correspond to specific organs, glands, and parts of the body. Stimulating these reflex points can promote relaxation, improve circulation, and support overall health and well-being.

2. Reflex Points: Specific points on the hands that correspond to different organs, glands, and parts of the body. By applying pressure to these points, reflexologists believe they can stimulate healing and balance in the corresponding areas of the body.

3. Meridians: In Traditional Chinese Medicine (TCM), meridians are energy pathways that run throughout the body. Stimulating specific points on the hands is believed to help restore balance and harmony to the body's energy flow along these meridians.

4. Zone Therapy: A form of reflexology that focuses on specific zones of the body. By stimulating reflex points within these zones, practitioners aim to promote healing and balance in the corresponding areas of the body.

5. Hasta Marma: In Ayurvedic medicine, hasta marma refers to the reflex points on the hands that correspond to different organs and systems in the body. Stimulating these points is believed to help balance the doshas (vata, pitta, and kapha) and promote overall health and well-being.

6. Marma Points: In Ayurvedic medicine, marma points are vital energy points located throughout the body. Stimulating marma points on the hands is believed to promote health and well-being by balancing the flow of prana (vital energy) in the body.

7. Digital Pressure: A technique used in reflexology where pressure is applied to the reflex points on the hands using the fingers and thumbs. This pressure is typically firm but gentle, and is applied in a rhythmic and systematic manner.

8. Hand Reflexology Chart: A visual representation of the reflex points on the hands and their corresponding areas of the body. Hand reflexology charts can vary in complexity, but typically show the major reflex points and their locations.

9. Energy Flow: The concept in reflexology that energy flows through the body along meridians or energy pathways. By stimulating reflex points on the hands, practitioners aim to improve the flow of energy and promote balance and harmony in the body.

10. Holistic Healing: The approach to health and wellness that considers the whole person—body, mind, and spirit. Reflexology is considered a holistic therapy because it aims to promote balance and well-being on all levels of the individual.

Comprehensive Index of Topics Covered in the "Hand Reflexology Compendium "

1. Introduction to Hand Reflexology

2. History and Origins of Hand Reflexology

3. Principles and Concepts of Hand Reflexology

4. Benefits of Hand Reflexology

5. How Hand Reflexology Works

6. Understanding Reflex Points on the Hands

7. Techniques Used in Hand Reflexology

8. Tools and Accessories for Hand Reflexology

9. Getting Started with Hand Reflexology

10. Preparing for a Hand Reflexology Session

11. Setting the Right Environment for Hand Reflexology

12. Techniques for Relaxation in Hand Reflexology

13. Mapping the Hands: Detailed Map of Reflex Points

14. How to Locate Reflex Points on the Hands

15. Understanding the Connection between Hands and Body

16. Practicing Hand Reflexology: Step-by-Step Guide

17. Common Hand Reflexology Techniques

18. Tips for Effective Hand Reflexology Sessions

19. Hand Reflexology for Specific Conditions

   - Pain Relief

   - Stress and Anxiety

   - Digestive Issues

   - Better Sleep

20. Incorporating Hand Reflexology into Your Wellness Routine

21. Integrating Hand Reflexology with Other Wellness Practices

22. Daily Hand Reflexology Exercises for Self-Care

23. Maintaining Hand Health for Reflexology

24. Advanced Hand Reflexology Techniques

25. Reflexology for Emotional Wellbeing through the Hands

26. Hand Reflexology for Energy Balance

27. Exploring Reflexology Traditions

   - Different Traditions and Approaches to Hand Reflexology

   - Cultural and Historical Perspectives

28. Troubleshooting Issues during Hand Reflexology Sessions

29. Future Trends and Innovations in Hand Reflexology

30. Glossary of Key Terms in Hand Reflexology

This comprehensive index covers a wide range of topics related to hand reflexology, providing readers with a thorough understanding of the practice and its benefits.

CONCLUSION

As you reach the end of "Hand Reflexology Compendium," you have embarked on a transformative journey, one that has opened your eyes to the remarkable healing potential of your hands. Throughout this comprehensive guide, you have learned the principles, techniques, and benefits of hand reflexology, empowering you to take charge of your health and well-being in a profound and meaningful way.

A Path to Wellness: Reflexology is more than just a therapeutic technique, it is a path to holistic wellness. By stimulating specific reflex points on your hands, you can alleviate pain, reduce stress, and promote healing throughout your body. Hand reflexology offers a natural, non-invasive approach to health that anyone can learn and practice, making it accessible to all.

Empowerment Through Knowledge: Armed with the knowledge and techniques provided in this book, you now have the power to enhance your health and well-being on a daily basis. Whether you are seeking relief from a specific ailment or simply looking to maintain your overall health, hand reflexology can be a valuable tool in your wellness arsenal.

A Lifetime of Benefits: As you continue to practice hand reflexology, you will discover a wealth of benefits that extend far beyond the physical. By incorporating hand reflexology into your daily routine, you can reduce stress, improve your mood, and enhance your overall quality of life. Your hands are not just instruments for daily tasks, they are powerful tools for promoting health, relieving stress, and enhancing your well-being.

The Journey Continues: Your journey with hand reflexology does not end here, it is a lifelong practice that can continue to enrich your life in countless ways. Whether you choose to practice hand reflexology for relaxation, pain relief, or simply to maintain your overall health, the benefits are endless.

Take the Next Step: As you close the pages of "Hand Reflexology Compendium," I encourage you to continue exploring the world of hand reflexology. Dive deeper into the practice, experiment with different techniques, and discover what works best for you. Your hands hold the key to a world of wellness, unlock their healing power and embrace a healthier, happier you.